The Complete Ketogenic Cooking Guide

Fit and Healthy Delicious Recipes To Live Healthy and Burn Fat

Michelle Lewis

2

Contents

Peanut butter sandwich chaffle

Preparation time: 15 minutes

Servings: 1

Ingredients: For chaffle:

1 egg, lightly beaten 1 tbsp swerve

1/2 cup mozzarella cheese, shredded

1/4 tsp espresso powder

1 tbsp unsweetened chocolate chips

2 tbsp unsweetened cocoa powder

For filling: 1 tbsp butter, softened

2 tbsp swerve 3 tbsp creamy peanut butter

Directions:

Preheat your waffle maker. In a bowl, whisk together egg, espresso powder, chocolate chips, swerve, and cocoa powder. Add mozzarella cheese and stir well. Spray waffle maker with Cooking spray. Pour 1/2 of the batter in the hot waffle maker and cook for 3-4 minutes or until golden brown. Repeat with the remaining batter. For filling: in a small bowl, stir together butter, swerve, and peanut butter until smooth. Once chaffles is cool, then spread filling mixture between two chaffle and place in the fridge for 10 minutes. Cut chaffle sandwich in half and Servings.

Nutrition:

Calories 190 Fat 16.1 g carbohydrates 9.6 g sugar 1.1 g
protein 8.2 g cholesterol 101 mg

Cherry chocolate chaffle

Preparation time: 10 minutes

Servings: 1

Ingredients:

1 egg, lightly beaten

1 tbsp unsweetened chocolate chips

2 tbsp sugar-free cherry pie fi lling

2 tbsp heavy whipping cream

1/2 cup mozzarella cheese, shredded

1/2 tsp baking powder, gluten-free

1 tbsp swerve

1 tbsp unsweetened cocoa powder

1 tbsp almond flour

Directions:

Preheat the waffle maker.

In a bowl, whisk together egg, cheese, baking powder, swerve, cocoa powder, and almond flour.

Spray waffle maker with Cooking spray.

Pour batter in the hot waffle maker and cook until golden brown.

Top with cherry pie filling, heavy whipping cream, and chocolate chips and Servings.

Nutrition: Calories 264 Fat 22 g carbohydrates 8.5 g sugar 0.5 g protein 12.7 g cholesterol 212 mg

Pumpkin chaffle with frosting

Preparation time: 15 minutes

Servings: 2

Ingredients: 1 egg, lightly beaten

1 tbsp sugar-free pumpkin puree

1/4 tsp pumpkin pie spice

1/2 cup mozzarella cheese, shredded

For frosting: 1/2 tsp vanilla 2 tbsp swerve

2 tbsp cream cheese, softened

Directions:

Preheat your waffle maker.

Add egg in a bowl and whisk well.

Add pumpkin puree, pumpkin pie spice, and cheese and stir well.

Spray waffle maker with Cooking spray.

Pour 1/2 of the batter in the hot waffle maker and cook for 3-4 minutes or until golden brown. Repeat with the remaining batter.

In a small bowl, mix all frosting Ingredients until smooth.

Add frosting on top of hot chaffles and Servings.

Nutrition:

Calories 98 Fat 7 g carbohydrates 3.6 g sugar 0.6 g protein 5.6 g cholesterol 97 mg

Breakfast peanut

butter chaffle

Preparation time: 15 minutes

Servings: 2

Ingredients:

1 egg, lightly beaten

½ tsp vanilla

1 tbsp swerve

2 tbsp powdered peanut butter

½ cup mozzarella cheese, shredded

Directions:

Preheat your waffle maker.

Add all Ingredients into the bowl and mix until well combined.

Spray waffle maker with Cooking spray.

Pour half batter in the hot waffle maker and cook for 5-7 minutes or until golden brown. Repeat with the remaining batter.

Servings and enjoy.

Nutrition:

Calories 80

Fat 4.1 g carbohydrates 2.9 g sugar 0.6 g protein 7.4 g cholesterol 86 mg

Wheat chaffles

Serving: 5 chaffles.

Preparation time: 10 minutes

Cooking time: 20 minutes

Ingredients

1 large egg, separated

3/4 cup milk

1/3 cup canola oil

1/4 cup orange juice

1 cup whole wheat flour

1 tablespoon sugar

1 to 1-1/2 teaspoons grated orange zest

1/2 cup mozzarella cheese, shredded

1 teaspoon baking powder

1/4 teaspoon salt

Direction

In a small bowl, beat the egg white until stiff peaks form; set aside. In another small bowl, beat egg yolk, milk, oil and orange juice. Combine flour, sugar, orange zest, baking powder and salt; stir into milk mixture. Add mozzarella cheese and stir well. Fold in egg white. Bake in a preheated waffle iron according to manufacturer's directions until golden brown.

Nutrition: Calories: 262 calories total fat: 17g cholesterol: 47mg sodium: 230mg total carbohydrate: 23g protein: 6g fiber: 3g

Whole grain chaffles with blackberry sauce

Serving: 4

Preparation time: 15 minutes

Cooking time: 15 minutes

Ingredients Cooking spray (such as pam®)

Batter: 2 cups whole wheat flour

2 cups milk 2 eggs

1/3 cup vegetable oil 1/2 teaspoon salt

1 tablespoon baking powder

1/2 cup mozzarella cheese, shredded

Blackberry sauce:

2 cups fresh blackberries 1/3 cup white sugar

2 tablespoons sifted cornstarch

1 tablespoon lemon juice

Direction

Preheat a waffle iron according to manufacturer's instructions. Prepare the Cooking surface with Cooking spray. Beat flour, milk, eggs, vegetable oil, baking powder, and salt together in a bowl using an electric mixer until batter is thoroughly mixed. Add mozzarella cheese and stir well. Pour about 1/4 cup batter per waffle into the preheated waffle iron and cook according to manufacturers' instructions. Stir blackberries together in a saucepan over high heat until heated through, 3 to 4 minutes. Decrease heat to medium and add sugar, cornstarch, and lemon juice to blackberries; cook and stir until sauce is thickened, about 5 minutes.

Nutrition: Calories: 575 calories total fat: 24.6 g cholesterol: 103 mg sodium: 746 mg total carbohydrate: 78 g protein: 16.4 g

Coconut chaffle

Preparation time: 5 minutes

Cooking time: 10 minutes

Servings: 4

Ingredients: ½ cup cream cheese, soft

1 tablespoon coconut flesh, unsweetened and shredded

2 teaspoons coconut oil, melted

1 tablespoon coconut flour 3 eggs, whisked

1 tablespoon erythritol

1 teaspoon vanilla extract

½ teaspoon almond extract

Directions:

In a bowl, combine the cream cheese with the melted coconut oil and the other Ingredients and whisk well. Heat up the waffle iron over high heat, pour ¼ of the batter, close the waffle maker, cook for 10 minutes and transfer to a plate. Repeat with the rest of the batter and Servings the chaffles warm.

Nutrition: calories 230, fat 11.2, fiber 1.2, carbs 3.4, protein 5.56

anilla raspberry chaffle

Preparation time: 5 minutes

ooking time: 8 minutes

Servings: 2

Ingredients:

½ cup cream cheese, soft

1 teaspoon vanilla extract

1 tablespoon almond flour

¼ cup raspberries, pureed

1 egg, whisked

1 tablespoon monk fruit

Directions:

In a bowl, mix the cream cheese with the raspberry puree and the other Ingredients and whisk well.

Heat up the waffle iron over high heat, pour half of the batter, close the waffle maker, cook for 8 minutes and transfer to a plate.

Repeat with the rest of the batter and Servings the chaffles warm.

Nutrition: calories 150, fat 9.3, fiber 1.2, carbs 3.4, protein 4.2

Nutmeg chaffle

Preparation time: 5 minutes

Cooking time: 5 minutes

Servings: 2

Ingredients:

3 tablespoons heavy cream

1 tablespoon coconut oil, melted

1 tablespoon coconut flour

1 egg, whisked

1 tablespoon stevia

½ teaspoon nutmeg, ground

2 tablespoons cream cheese

½ teaspoon vanilla extract

Directions:

In a bowl, mix the cream with the coconut oil, egg and the other Ingredients and whisk well.

Heat up the waffle iron over high heat, pour half of the batter, close the waffle maker, cook for 5 minutes and transfer to a plate.

Repeat with the remaining batter and Servings.

Nutrition: calories 200, fat 15, fiber 1.2, carbs 3.4, protein 12.05

Almond plums chaffle

Preparation time: 5 minutes

Cooking time: 6 minutes Servings: 4

Ingredients:

½ cup heavy cream

½ cup almonds, chopped

2 plums, pitted and chopped

1 tablespoon almond flour

3 eggs, whisked

2 tablespoons erythritol

2 tablespoons cream cheese

Directions:

In a bowl, mix the cream with the almonds, plums and the other Ingredients and whisk well.

Heat up the waffle iron over high heat, pour ¼ of the batter, close the waffle maker, cook for 6 minutes and transfer to a plate.

Repeat with the remaining batter and Servings the chaffles warm.

Nutrition: calories 220, fat 13.25, fiber 1.2, carbs 5.4, protein 12

Almond butter chaffle

Preparation time: 5 minutes

Cooking time: 6 minutes

Servings: 4

Ingr edients:

4 eggs, whisked

1 cup almond flour

2 tablespoons swerve

½ cup almond butter, soft

1 teaspoon baking soda

2 teaspoons vanilla extract

2 tablespoons coconut oil, melted

Directions:

In a bowl, combine the eggs with the almond flour, swerve and the other Ingredients and whisk well.

Heat up the waffle iron over high heat, pour ¼ of the batter, close the waffle maker, cook for 6 minutes and transfer to a plate.

Repeat with the rest batter and Servings the chaffles warm.

Nutrition: calories 220, fat 4.3, fiber 1.2, carbs 3.4, protein 7.5

int chaffle

Preparation time: 5 minutes

Cooking time: 5 minutes

Servings: 2

Ingredients:

½ cup cream cheese, soft

1 tablespoon almond flour

½ tablespoon coconut flour

2 eggs whisked

1 tablespoon swerve

2 tablespoons mint, chopped

1 teaspoon vanilla extract

½ teaspoon almond extract

Directions:

In a bowl, combine the cream cheese with the flour and the other Ingredients and whisk well.

Heat up the waffle iron over high heat, pour half of the batter, close the waffle maker, cook for 5 minutes and transfer to a plate.

Repeat with the other part of the batter and Servings the chaffles warm.

Nutrition: calories 182, fat 8.3, fiber 1.2, carbs 3.4, protein 6.5

Melon puree chaffle

Preparation time: 5 minutes

Cooking time: 5 minutes

Servings: 2

Ingredients:

½ cup melon, peeled and pureed

3 tablespoons cream cheese, soft

1 tablespoon coconut flour

1 egg, whisked

1 tablespoon stevia

½ teaspoon almond extract

Directions:

In a bowl, mix the melon puree with the cream cheese and the other Ingredients and whisk well.

Heat up the waffle iron over high heat, pour half of the batter, close the waffle maker, cook for 5 minutes and transfer to a plate.

Repeat with the other part of the batter and Servings.

Nutrition: calories 252, fat 14.3, fiber 3.2, carbs 4.4, protein 2.3

Sweet zucchini chaffle

Preparation time: 5 minutes

Cooking time: 7 minutes

Servings: 4

Ingredients:

½ cup zucchinis, grated

4 tablespoons cream cheese, soft

1 tablespoon almond flour

1 tablespoon almonds, chopped

2 eggs, whisked

1 tablespoon swerve

½ teaspoon vanilla extract

Directions:

In a bowl, mix the zucchinis with the cream cheese, almond flour and other Ingredients and whisk well.

Heat up the waffle iron over high heat, pour ¼ of the batter, close the waffle maker, cook for 7 minutes and transfer to a plate.

Repeat with the remaining batter and Servings the chaffles hot.

Nutrition: calories 220, fat 12.4, fiber 2.2, carbs 3.4, protein 6.4

Pumpkin and avocado chaffle

Preparation time: 5 minutes

Cooking time: 5 minutes

Servings: 4

Ingredients:

½ cup heavy cream

1 avocado, peeled, pitted and mashed

1 tablespoon coconut flour

2 eggs, whisked

2 tablespoons swerve

2 and ½ tablespoons pumpkin puree

2 tablespoons cream cheese, soft

Directions:

In a bowl, combine the cream with the avocado, pumpkin puree and the other Ingredients and whisk.

Heat up the waffle iron over high heat, pour ¼ of the batter, close the waffle maker, cook for 5 minutes and transfer to a plate.

Repeat with the rest of the batter and Servings the chaffles warm.

Nutrition: calories 220, fat 9.4, fiber 1.2, carbs 3, protein 7.6

Nuts chaffle

Preparation time: 5 minutes

Cooking time: 8 minutes

Servings: 4

Ingredients:

2 tablespoons almonds, chopped

2 tablespoons walnuts, chopped

1 tablespoon stevia

½ cup cream cheese, soft

2 eggs, whisked

1 tablespoon almond flour

1 tablespoon coconut flour

½ teaspoon almond extract

Directions:

In a blender, mix the almonds with the walnuts, cream cheese and the other Ingredients and pulse well.

Heat up the waffle iron over high heat, pour ¼ of the batter, close the waffle maker, cook for 5 minutes and transfer to a plate.

Repeat with the other part of the batter and Servings.

Nutrition: calories 200, fat 9.34, fiber 2.2, carbs 4.4, protein 8.4

Blueberries and

almonds chaffles

Preparation time: 5 minutes

Cooking time: 8 minutes

Servings: 6

Ingredients:

½ cup cream cheese, soft

½ cup blueberries pureed

2 tablespoons almonds

1 tablespoon almond flour

2 eggs, whisked

1 and ½ tablespoon stevia

½ teaspoon almond extract

Directions:

In a bowl, mix the cream cheese with the blueberries, eggs and the other Ingredients and whisk well.

Heat up the waffle iron over high heat, pour 1/6 of the batter, close the waffle maker, cook for 5 minutes and transfer to a plate.

Repeat with the other part of the batter and Servings.

Nutrition: calories 180, fat 5.4, fiber 1.2, carbs 2.24, protein 2.4

Rhubarb chaffles

Preparation time: 5 minutes

Cooking time: 6 minutes

Servings: 3

Ingredients:

½ cup rhubarb, chopped

¼ cup heavy cream

3 tablespoons cream cheese, soft

2 tablespoons almond flour

2 eggs, whisked

2 tablespoons swerve

½ teaspoon vanilla extract

½ teaspoon nutmeg, ground

Directions:

In a bowl, mix the rhubarb with the cream, cream cheese and the other Ingredients and whisk well.

Heat up the waffle iron over high heat, pour 1/3 of the batter, close the waffle maker, cook for 5 minutes and transfer to a plate.

Repeat with the rest of the chaffle batter and Servings.

Nutrition: calories 180, fat 4, fiber 1.2, carbs 2, protein 2.4

Sweet turmeric chaffles

Preparation time: 5 minutes

Cooking time: 6 minutes

Servings: 2

Ingredients:

3 tablespoons cream cheese, soft

½ teaspoon turmeric powder

½ teaspoon vanilla extract

2 tablespoons coconut flour

2 eggs, whisked

2 tablespoons stevia

Directions:

In a bowl, mix the cream cheese with the turmeric, vanilla and the other Ingredients and whisk well.

Heat up the waffle iron over high heat, pour ½ of the batter, close the waffle maker, cook for 6 minutes and transfer to a plate.

Repeat with the other part of the batter and Servings right away.

Nutrition: calories 140, fat 4.4, fiber 1.2, carbs 5.4, protein 4.4

Banana pudding chaffle cake

Preparation time: 5 minutes

Cooking time: 5 minutes

Servings: 2

Ingredients 1 large egg yolk

1/2 cup fresh cream 3 t powder sweetener

1 4-1 2 teaspoon xanthan gum

1/2 teaspoon banana extract

Banana chaffle Ingredients

1 oz softened cream cheese

1/4 cup mozzarella cheese shredded

1 egg 1 teaspoon banana extract

2 t sweetener 1 tsp baking powder

4 t almond flour

Preparations

Mix heavy cream, powdered sweetener and egg yolk in a small pot. Whisk constantly until the sweetener has dissolved and the mixture is thick. Cook for 1 minute. Add xanthan gum and whisk. Remove from heat, add a pinch of salt and banana extract and stir well. Transfer to a glass dish and cover the pudding with plastic wrap. Refrigerate.Mix all Ingredients together. Cook in a preheated mini waffle maker.

Note

Make three chaffles. 3.3 net carbs / serving. Recipe 9.8 net carbs nutritional value

Maple Pumpkin Ketogenic Chaffle

Preparation time: 5 *Minutes*

Cooking Time : 4 *Minutes*

Servings: 2

Ingredients 3/4 tsp baking powder

2 eggs 4 tsp heavy whipping cream

1/2 cup mozzarella cheese, shredded

2 tsp Liquid Stevia

Pinch of salt

3/4 tsp pumpkin pie spice 1 tsp coconut flour

2 tsp pumpkin puree (100% pumpkin)

1/2 tsp vanilla

Directions

Preheat mini waffle maker until hot Whisk egg in a bowl, add cheese, then mix well Stir in the remaining Ingredients (except toppings, if any).Scoop 1/2 of the batter onto the waffle maker, spread across evenly Cook 3-4 minutes, until done as desired (or crispy). Gently remove from waffle maker and let it cool Repeat with remaining batter. Top with sugar-free maple syrup or Ketogenic ice cream.

Servings and Enjoy!

Nutrition: 201 calories 2g net carbs 15g fat 12g protein

Ketogenic Almond

Blueberry Chaffle

Preparation time: 5 Minutes

Cooking Time: 5 Minutes

Servings: 5 Chaffles

Ingredients 1 tsp baking powder

2 eggs 1 cup of mozzarella cheese

2 tablespoons almond flour

3 tablespoon blueberries 1 tsp cinnamon

2 tsp of Swerve

Directions

Preheat mini waffle maker until hot Whisk egg in a bowl, add cheese, then mix well Stir in the remaining Ingredients (except toppings, if any). Grease the preheated waffle maker with non-stick Cooking spray. Scoop 1/2 of the batter onto the waffle maker, spread across evenly Cook until a bit browned and crispy, about 4 minutes. Cook 3-4 minutes, until done as desired (or crispy). Gently remove from waffle maker and let it cool

Repeat with remaining batter.

Top with Ketogenic syrup

Servings and Enjoy!

Nutrition: 116 calories 1g net carbs 8g fat 8g protein

Sweet Cinnamon

"Sugar" Chaffle

Preparation time: 5 *Minutes*

Cooking Time : 4 *Minutes*

Servings: 1

Ingredients 1/2 teaspoon cinnamon (topping)

10 drops of liquid stevia

1 tablespoon almond flour

Two large eggs

A splash of vanilla 1/2 cup mozzarella cheese

Directions

Preheat waffle maker until hot

Whisk egg in a bowl, add cheese, then mix well Stir in the remaining Ingredients (except toppings, if any).

Scoop 1/2 of the batter onto the waffle maker, spread across evenly

Cook 3-4 minutes, until done as desired (or crispy). Gently remove from waffle maker and let it cool

Repeat with remaining batter.

Top with melted butter and sprinkle of cinnamon.

Servings and Enjoy!

Nutrition: 221 calories 2g net carbs 17g fat 12g protein

Chocolatey Chaffle

Preparation time: 5 *Minutes*

Cooking Time : 4 *Minutes*

Servings: 2

Ingredients: 1 large egg

1 oz. cream cheese, softened

1 tbsp ChocZero Chocolate Syrup

1/2 tsp vanilla 1 tbsp Stevia sweetener

1/2 tbsp cacao powder

1/4 tsp baking powder

Directions

Preheat mini waffle maker until hot

Whisk egg in a bowl, add cheese, then mix well

Stir in the remaining Ingredients (except toppings, if any).

Scoop 1/2 of the batter onto the waffle maker, spread across evenly

Cook until a bit browned and crispy, about 4 minutes.

Gently remove from waffle maker and let it cool

Repeat with remaining batter.

Servings and Enjoy!

Nutrition: 241 calories 2g net carbs 19g fat 13g protein

Ketogenic Chocolate Chip Chaffle

Preparation time: 5 *Minutes*

Cooking Time : 8 *Minutes*

Servings: 1

Ingredients 1 egg 1/4 tsp baking powder

Pinch of salt

1 tbsp heavy whipping cream (topping)

1/2 tsp coconut flour 1 tbsp Chocolate Chips

Directions

Preheat mini waffle maker until hot Whisk egg in a bowl, add cheese, then mix well

Stir in the remaining Ingredients (except toppings, if any). Grease preheated waffle maker with. This will help to create a more crisp crust. Scoop 1/2 of the batter onto the waffle maker, spread across evenly.

Sprinkle chocolate chips on top

Cook until a bit browned and crispy, about 4 minutes.

Gently remove from waffle maker and let it cool

Repeat with remaining batter.

Top with whipping cream

Servings and Enjoy!

Nutrition: 146 calories 3g net carbs 10g fat 6g protein

Pumpkin Chocolate

Chip Chaffles

Preparation time: 4 *Minutes*

Cooking Time : 12 *Minutes*

Servings: 3

Ingredients 2 tbsp granulated swerve

1/4 tsp pumpkin pie spice

1 tbsp almond flour

1/2 cup shredded mozzarella cheese

4 tsp pumpkin puree 1 egg

4 tsp chocolate chips

Directions

Preheat mini waffle maker until hot Whisk egg in a bowl, add cheese, then mix well Stir in the remaining Ingredients (except toppings, if any). Grease waffle maker and Scoop 1/2 of the batter onto the waffle maker, spread across evenly. Add chocolate chips on top the batter and cook until a bit browned and crispy, about 4 minutes.

Gently remove from waffle maker and let it cool Repeat with remaining batter.

Servings and Enjoy with some cream!

Nutrition: 93 calories 1g net carbs 7g fat 7g protein

Mint Chocolate Chaffle

Preparation time: 5 *Minutes*

Cooking Time : 4 *Minutes*

Servings: 2

Ingredients: 1 large egg

1 oz. cream cheese, softened

1 tbsp chocolate chips 1 tbsp Stevia sweetener

1 tbsp low carb mint extract

1/2 tbsp cacao powder

1/4 tsp baking powder

Directions

Preheat mini waffle maker until hot

Whisk egg in a bowl, add cheese, then mix well

Stir in the remaining Ingredients (except toppings, if any).

Scoop 1/2 of the batter onto the waffle maker, spread across evenly

Cook until a bit browned and crispy, about 4 minutes.

Gently remove from waffle maker and let it cool

Repeat with remaining batter.

Servings and Enjoy!

Nutrition: 241 calories 2g net carbs 19g fat 13g protein

Ketogenic Coco-Chaffle

Preparation time: 5 *Minutes*

Cooking Time : 8 *Minutes*

Servings: 1

Ingredients 1 egg 1/4 tsp baking powder

Pinch of salt

1 tbsp heavy whipping cream (topping)

1/2 tsp coconut flour

1 tbsp Chocolate Chips

Directions

Preheat mini waffle maker until hot Whisk egg in a bowl, add cheese, then mix well Stir in the remaining Ingredients (except toppings, if any).

Grease preheated waffle maker with non-stick Cooking spray. Scoop 1/2 of the batter onto the waffle maker, spread across evenly.

Sprinkle cocoa powder on top

Cook until a bit browned and crispy, about 4 minutes.

Gently remove from waffle maker and let it cool Repeat with remaining batter.

Top with whipping cream

Servings and Enjoy!

Nutrition: 146 calories 3g net carbs 10g fat 6g protein

Ketogenic Vanilla Brownie Chaffle

Preparation time: 5 *Minutes*

Cooking Time : 4 *Minutes*

Servings: 2

Ingredients: 1 large egg

1 oz. cream cheese, softened

1 tbsp ChocZero Chocolate Syrup

1/2 tsp vanilla 2 tbsp Stevia sweetener

2 tbsp cacao powder

1/4 tsp baking powder

Directions

Preheat mini waffle maker until hot

Whisk egg in a bowl, add cheese, then mix well

Stir in the remaining Ingredients (except toppings, if any).

Scoop 1/2 of the batter onto the waffle maker, spread across evenly

Cook until a bit browned and crispy, about 4 minutes.

Gently remove from waffle maker and let it cool

Repeat with remaining batter. Servings and Enjoy with topped melted butter!

Nutrition: 241 calories 2g net carbs 19g fat 13g protein

Ketogenic Crispy Choco Chaffle

Preparation time: 5 *Minutes*

Cooking Time : 8 *Minutes*

Servings: 1

Ingredients 1 egg 1/4 tsp baking powder

Pinch of salt

1 tbsp almond butter (topping)

1/2 tsp almond flour

1 tbsp Chocolate Chips

1 tsp cheddar cheese (Servings ½ for greasing)

Directions

Preheat mini waffle maker until hot Whisk egg in a bowl, add cheese, then mix well Stir in the remaining Ingredients (except toppings, if any). Grease preheated waffle maker with 1 tsp of shredded cheese. Cook for 20 seconds. This will help to create a more crisp crust. Scoop 1/2 of the batter onto the waffle maker, spread across evenly. Sprinkle chocolate chips on top Cook until a bit browned and crispy, about 4 minutes. Gently remove from waffle maker and let it cool Repeat with remaining batter.

Top with whipping cream

Servings and Enjoy!

Nutrition: 146 calories 3g net carbs 10g fat 6g protein

Almond Chocolate Chaffle

Preparation time: 5 *Minutes*

Cooking Time : 4 *Minutes*

Servings: 2

Ingredients: 1 large egg

1 oz. cream cheese, softened

1 tbsp ChocZero Chocolate Syrup

1/2 tsp vanilla 1 tbsp Stevia sweetener

1/2 tbsp cacao powder

1/4 tsp baking powder

One handful almond nuts, cut in bit sizes (topping)

Directions

 Preheat mini waffle maker until hot Whisk egg in a bowl, add cheese, then mix well Stir in the remaining Ingredients (except toppings). Scoop 1/2 of the batter onto the waffle maker, spread across evenly Sprinkle Almond nuts, then cover and Cook until a bit browned and crispy, about 4 minutes.

Gently remove from waffle maker and let it cool

Repeat with remaining batter.

Servings and Enjoy!

Nutrition: 241 calories 2g net carbs 19g fat 13g protein

Ketogenic Chocolate Chip Chaffle

Preparation time: 5 *Minutes*

Cooking Time : 8 *Minutes*

Servings: 1

Ingredients 1 egg

1/4 tsp baking powder

Pinch of salt

1 tbsp cinnamon (topping)

1/2 tsp coconut flour

1 tbsp Chocolate Chips

Directions

Preheat mini waffle maker until hot

Whisk egg in a bowl, add cheese, then mix well Stir in the remaining Ingredients (except toppings, if any). Grease preheated waffle maker with. This will help to create a more crisp crust.

Scoop 1/2 of the batter onto the waffle maker, spread across evenly.

Sprinkle chocolate chips on top

Cook until a bit browned and crispy, about 4 minutes. Gently remove from waffle maker and let it cool Repeat with remaining batter.

Top with whipping cream

Servings and Enjoy!

Nutrition: 146 calories 3g net carbs 10g fat 6g protein

Sweet Raspberry Chaffle

Preparation time: 5 Minutes

Cooking Time: 5 Minutes

Servings: 5 Chaffles

Ingredients

1 tsp baking powder

2 eggs

1 cup of mozzarella cheese

2 tbsp almond flour

4 raspberries, chopped

1 tsp cinnamon

10 drops Stevia, liquid

Directions

Preheat mini waffle maker until hot

Whisk egg in a bowl, add cheese, then mix well Stir in the remaining Ingredients (except toppings, if any). Grease the preheated waffle maker with non-stick Cooking spray. Scoop 1/2 of the batter onto the waffle maker, spread across evenly Cook until a bit browned and crispy, about 4 minutes. Cook 3-4 minutes, until done as desired (or crispy). Gently remove from waffle maker and let it cool Repeat with remaining batter. Top with Ketogenic syrup Servings and Enjoy!

Nutrition: 116 calories 1g net carbs 8g fat 8g protein

Avocado pizza chaffle

Preparation time: 5 minutes

Cooking time: 6 minutes

Servings: 2

Ingredients: 2 eggs, whisked

½ cup cream cheese, soft

1 avocado, peeled, pitted and cubed

1 teaspoon garam masala

2 tablespoons cheddar, grated

2 tablespoons tomato passata

Directions:

In a bowl, mix the eggs with the cream cheese and garam masala and whisk well. Preheat the waffle iron over medium-high heat, pour half of the chaffle mix, cook for 6 minutes and transfer to a plate. Repeat with the remaining of the batter, divide the passata, avocado and cheddar over the chaffles and Servings.

Nutrition: calories 252, fat 8.3, fiber 4.2, carbs 5, protein 11.2

Kale and chicken chaffle

Preparation time: 5 minutes

Cooking time: 6 minutes

Servings: 3

Ingredients: 2 eggs, whisked

½ cup baby kale, torn

½ cup mozzarella, shredded

¼ cup cream cheese

¼ cup chicken breast, skinless, cooked and shredded ½ teaspoon garlic powder

2 tablespoons tomato passata

Directions:

In a bowl, mix the eggs with half of the mozzarella, cream cheese and garlic powder and stir. Preheat the waffle iron over medium-high heat, pour 1/3 of the chaffle mix, cook for 6 minutes and transfer to a plate.

Repeat with the rest of the batter, spread the passata over the chaffles, divide the kale and chicken and Servings.

Nutrition: calories 302, fat 8.3, fiber 4.2, carbs 5, protein 18

Kale and mushroom chaffle

Preparation time: 5 minutes

Cooking time: 6 minutes

Servings: 2

Ingredients:

2 eggs, whisked

3 tablespoons cream cheese, soft

2 tablespoons heavy cream

½ cup baby kale, torn

¼ cup mushrooms, sliced

1 tablespoon cheddar, shredded

2 tablespoons tomato passata

Directions:

In a bowl, mix the eggs with the cream cheese and cream and stir.

Preheat the waffle iron over medium-high heat, pour half of the chaffle mix, cook for 6 minutes and transfer to a plate.

Repeat with the rest of the batter, sprinkle the passata, kale, mushrooms and cheddar over the chaffles and Servings.

Nutrition: calories 302, fat 9.3, fiber 4.2, carbs 5, protein 11

Pepperoni pizza chaffle

Preparation time: 5 minutes

Cooking time: 7 minutes

Servings: 4

Ingredients:

3 eggs, whisked

½ cup mozzarella, shredded

½ cup cream cheese, soft

½ tablespoon butter, melted

2 tablespoons cheddar, shredded

½ cup pepperoni, sliced

2 tablespoons capers, drained

1 tablespoon black olives, pitted and sliced

3 tablespoons tomato passata

Directions:

In a bowl, mix the eggs with the mozzarella, cream cheese and melted butter and stir well.

Preheat the waffle iron over medium-high heat, pour ¼ of the chaffle mix, cook for 7 minutes and transfer to a plate.

Repeat with the rest of the batter, spread the passata over them, sprinkle the cheddar, capers and the other over the chaffles and Servings.

Nutrition: calories 322, fat 11.3, fiber 2.2, carbs 5, protein 9.2

Asparagus pizza chaffle

Preparation time: 5 minutes

Cooking time: 5 minutes

Servings: 2

Ingredients:

2 eggs, whisked

½ cup asparagus, chopped

2 scallions, chopped

½ cup cream cheese, soft

½ cup mozzarella, shredded

½ teaspoon turmeric powder

½ teaspoon garam masala

2 tablespoons tomato passata

Directions:

In a bowl, mix the eggs with the cream cheese, mozzarella, turmeric and garam masala and stir well.

Preheat the waffle iron over medium-high heat, pour half of the chaffle mix, cook for 6 minutes and transfer to a plate.

Repeat with the rest of the batter, spread the passata over the chaffles, sprinkle the remaining Ingredients and Servings warm.

Nutrition: calories 252, fat 8.3, fiber 4.2, carbs 5, protein 11.2

Salmon pizza chaffle

Preparation time: 5 minutes

Cooking time: 6 minutes

Servings: 4

Ingredients:

3 eggs, whisked

½ cup mozzarella, shredded

3 tablespoons heavy cream

½ cup smoked salmon, skinless, boneless and flaked

½ cup baby spinach, torn

½ cup cherry tomatoes, cubed

2 tablespoons cream cheese, soft

3 tablespoons tomato passata

Directions:

In a bowl, mix the eggs with the cheese, cream and cream cheese and stir well.

Preheat the waffle iron over medium-high heat, pour ¼ of the chaffle mix, cook for 6 minutes and transfer to a plate.

Repeat with the rest of the batter, spread the passata over the chaffles, divide the salmon and the other Ingredients and Servings.

Nutrition: calories 272, fat 5.3, fiber 2.2, carbs 3, protein 7

Tuna pizza chaffle

Preparation time: 5 minutes

Cooking time: 8 minutes

Servings: 4

Ingredients:

½ cup canned tuna, drained and flaked

3 eggs, whisked

½ cup mozzarella, shredded

1 teaspoon sweet paprika

½ teaspoon rosemary, dried

2 tablespoons spring onions, chopped

1 tablespoon cilantro, chopped

2 tablespoons cream cheese, soft

¼ cup spinach, torn

3 tablespoons tomato passata

Directions:

In a bowl, mix the eggs with the cheese, paprika, rosemary, and cream cheese and stir well.

Preheat the waffle iron over medium-high heat, pour ¼ of the chaffle mix, cook for 8 minutes and transfer to a plate.

Repeat with the rest of the batter, spread the passata over the chaffles, divide the tuna and the remaining Ingredients and Servings.

Nutrition: calories 310, fat 11.3, fiber4.2, carbs 5, protein 7.6Ketogenic Pizza Chaffle

Preparation time: 5 *Minutes*

Cooking Time : 4 *Minutes*

Servings: 2

Ingredients: 1 egg 1/2 cup mozzarella cheese, shredded Just a pinch of Italian seasoning 1 tbsp Pizza sauce (without added sugar) Shredded cheese, and pepperoni (or any favorite toppings) Instructions:

Preheat mini waffle maker until hot

Whisk egg in a bowl, add cheese, then mix well

Stir in the remaining Ingredients (except toppings, if any).

Add a bit of shredded cheese to the preheated waffle maker. Let it cook for 20 seconds. This will help to create a more crisp crust.

Scoop 1/2 of the batter onto the waffle maker, spread across evenly

Cook until a bit browned and crispy, about 4 minutes.

Gently remove from waffle maker and let it cool

Repeat with remaining batter.

Top with pizza sauce, shredded cheese, and pepperoni. Microwave on high for 20 seconds

Servings and Enjoy!

Nutrition: 219 calories 2g net carbs 22g fat 12g protein

Delicious Pizza Chaffle Recipe

Preparation time: 5 *Minutes*

Cooking Time : 15 *Minutes*

Servings: 2

Ingredients 1 egg white Pinch of salt 1 tsp cream cheese, softened 1 tbsp parmesan cheese, shredded 1/8 tsp garlic powder 1/2 cup mozzarella cheese, shredded 1/4 tsp basil seasoning 1/2 cup mozzarella cheese 6 pepperonis cut in half 1/8 tsp Italian seasoning 3 tsp low carb marinara sauce 1/4 tsp baking powder 1 tsp coconut flour

Instructions

Preheat waffle maker until hot Whisk egg in a bowl, add cheese, then mix well

Stir in the remaining Ingredients (except toppings, if any). Add a bit of cheese to the preheated waffle maker. This will help to create a more crisp crust.

Scoop 1/2 of the batter onto the waffle maker, spread across evenly Top with pepperoni, tomato sauce, and mozzarella and parmesan cheese. Microwave on high for 20 seconds Cook 3-4 minutes, until done as desired (or crispy). Gently remove from waffle maker and let it cool Repeat with remaining batter. Servings and Enjoy!

Nutrition: 241 calories 2g net carbs 18g fat 17g protein

Spicy Pizza Chaffle

Preparation time: 5 *Minutes*

Cooking Time : 4 *Minutes*

Servings: 2

Ingredients: 1 egg 1/2 cup mozzarella cheese, shredded A pinch of low carb seasoning mix 1 tbsp Pizza sauce (without added sugar) ¼ tsp kosher salt 1/2 cup heavy whipping cream (for topping) Shredded cheese, and pepperoni (for toppings) 1/2 tbsp Jalapenos slices (for topping)

Instructions:

Preheat mini waffle maker until hot Whisk egg in a bowl, add cheese, then mix well Stir in the remaining Ingredients (except toppings, if any). Add a bit of shredded cheese to the preheated waffle maker. Let it cook for 20 seconds. This will help to create a more crisp crust. Scoop 1/2 of the batter onto the waffle maker, spread across evenly

Cook until a bit browned and crispy, about 4 minutes. Gently remove from waffle maker and let it cool

Repeat with remaining batter.

Top with pizza sauce, shredded cheese, jalapenos and pepperoni. Microwave on high for 20 seconds Servings and Enjoy!

Nutrition: 219 calories 2g net carbs 22g fat 12g protein

Cheezy Pizza Chaffle

Preparation time: 5 *Minutes*

Cooking Time : 15 *Minutes*

Servings: 2

Ingredients 1 egg white Pinch of salt 1 tsp cream cheese, softened 1 tbsp parmesan cheese, shredded 1/8 tsp garlic powder 1/2 cup mozzarella cheese, shredded 1/4 tsp basil seasoning 1/2 cup mozzarella cheese 6 pepperonis cut in half 1/8 tsp Italian seasoning 3 tsp low carb marinara sauce 1/4 tsp baking powder 1 tsp coconut flour

Instructions

Preheat waffle maker until hot Whisk egg in a bowl, add cheese, then mix well Stir in the remaining Ingredients (except toppings, if any). Add a bit of cheese to the preheated waffle maker. This will help to create a more crisp crust.

Scoop 1/2 of the batter onto the waffle maker, spread across evenly Top with pepperoni, tomato sauce, and mozzarella and parmesan cheese. Microwave on high for 20 seconds Cook 3-4 minutes, until done as desired (or crispy). Gently remove from waffle maker and let it cool

Repeat with remaining batter.

Servings and Enjoy!

Nutrition: 241 calories 2g net carbs 18g fat 17g protein

Low Carb Pizza Chaffle Cups

Preparation time: 5 *Minutes*

Cooking Time : 4 *Minutes*

Servings: 2

Ingredients: 1 egg 1/2 cup mozzarella cheese, shredded Just a pinch of Italian seasoning 1 tbsp Pizza sauce (without added sugar) Shredded cheese, and pepperoni (or any favorite toppings)

Instructions:

Preheat mini waffle maker until hot

Whisk egg in a bowl, add cheese, then mix well Stir in the remaining Ingredients (except toppings, if any).

Add a bit of shredded cheese to the preheated waffle maker. Let it cook for 20 seconds. This will help to create a more crisp crust.

Scoop 1/2 of the batter onto the waffle maker, spread across evenly

Cook until a bit browned and crispy, about 4 minutes. Gently remove from waffle maker and let it cool Repeat with remaining batter.

Top with pizza sauce, shredded cheese, and pepperoni. Microwave on high for 20 seconds

Servings and Enjoy!

Nutrition: 219 calories 2g net carbs 22g fat 12g protein

Crispy Pizza Chaffle

Preparation time: 5 *Minutes*

Cooking Time : 15 *Minutes*

Servings: 2

Ingredients 1 egg white Pinch of salt 1 tsp cream cheese, softened 1/8 tsp garlic powder 1/2 cup mozzarella cheese, shredded 1/4 tsp basil seasoning 1/2 cup mozzarella cheese 4 pepperonis cut in half 1/4 tsp Italian seasoning 2 tsp low carb marinara sauce 1/4 tsp baking powder 1 tsp Psyllium husk powder (for added texture) Instructions

Preheat waffle maker until hot

Whisk egg in a bowl, add cheese, then mix well

Stir in the remaining Ingredients (except toppings, if any).

Add a bit of cheese to the preheated waffle maker. This will help to create a more crisp crust.

Scoop 1/2 of the batter onto the waffle maker, spread across evenly

Top with pepperoni, tomato sauce, and mozzarella and parmesan cheese. Microwave on high for 20 seconds

Cook 3-4 minutes, until done as desired (or crispy).

Gently remove from waffle maker and let it cool

Repeat with remaining batter.

Servings and Enjoy!

Nutrition: 241 calories 2g net carbs 18g fat 17g protein

Habanero chaffles

Preparation time: 10 minutes

Cooking time: 6 minutes

Servings: 4

Ingredients: 2 eggs, whisked

1 cup roasted red peppers, chopped

1 habanero pepper, minced

1 cup mozzarella, shredded

½ cup almond milk

1 teaspoon smoked paprika

1 tablespoon cilantro, chopped

½ teaspoon baking powder

Directions:

In a bowl, mix the eggs with the roasted peppers, habanero and the other Ingredients and whisk well. Preheat the waffle maker, pour ¼ of the batter, cook for 6 minutes and transfer to a plate.

Repeat with the rest of the batter and Servings.

Nutrition: calories 220, fat 4, fiber 2, carbs 5.3, protein 5.6

Hot salsa chaffles

Preparation time: 10 minutes

Cooking time: 7 minutes

Servings: 4

Ingredients:1 cup almond milk

1 cup almond flour ½ cup hot salsa

2 tablespoons ghee, melted 2 eggs, whisked

1 teaspoon baking soda

½ cup mozzarella, shredded

A pinch of salt and black pepper

½ cup chives, chopped

Directions:

In a bowl, mix the milk with the flour, salsa and the other Ingredients and whisk really well. Heat up the waffle iron, pour ¼ of the batter, cook for 7 minutes and transfer to a plate. Repeat with the rest of the salsa chaffle mix and Servings.

Nutrition: calories 262, fat 8, fiber 2.4, carbs 3.2, protein 8

Chili paste chaffles

Preparation time: 10 minutes

Cooking time: 8 minutes

Servings: 4

Ingredients:

1 cup coconut flour

1 cup water

1 tablespoon chili paste

2 eggs, whisked

½ cup parmesan, grated

1 teaspoon chili powder

A pinch of salt and black pepper

1 teaspoon baking soda

Directions:

In a bowl mix the flour with the water, chili paste and the other Ingredients and whisk well.

Heat up the waffle iron, pour ¼ of the batter, cook for 8 minutes, transfer to a platter, repeat with the rest of the mix and Servings.

Nutrition: calories 272, fat 9.4, fiber 2.3, carbs 4, protein 4

Hot BBQ chaffles

Preparation time: 10 minutes

Cooking time: 10 minutes

Servings: 6

Ingredients:

1 cup coconut flour

1 cup warm water

½ cup cheddar cheese, shredded

½ cup bbq sauce

1 teaspoon chili powder

1 teaspoon hot paprika

1 tablespoon spring onions, chopped

2 scallions, chopped

2 teaspoons baking powder

2 eggs, whisked

1 teaspoon cayenne pepper

Directions:

In a bowl, mix the flour with the water, bbq sauce and the
other Ingredients and whisk well. Preheat the waffle iron,

pour 1/6 of the batter, cook for 10 minutes and transfer to a plate. Repeat with the rest of the batter and Servings.

Nutrition: calories 292, fat 7, fiber 2.3, carbs 5, protein 8

Chili oil chaffles

Preparation time: 10 minutes

Cooking time: 8 minutes

Servings: 4

Ingredients:

2 eggs, whisked

1 cup spring onions, chopped

1 cup mozzarella, shredded

½ cup coconut milk

1 tablespoon chili olive oil

1 teaspoon chili powder

½ teaspoon parsley flakes, ground

Directions:

In a bowl, mix the eggs with the spring onions, mozzarella and the other Ingredients and whisk well.

Preheat the waffle iron, pour ¼ of the batter, cook for 8 minutes and transfer to a plate.

Repeat with the rest of the batter and Servings.

Nutrition: calories 260, fat 8.2, fiber 2.2, carbs 5.3, protein 12

Red pepper chaffles

Preparation time: 10 minutes

Cooking time: 6 minutes

Servings: 4

Ingredients:

1 cup almond flour

½ cup cream cheese, soft

½ cup coconut milk

1 teaspoon red pepper, crushed

2 green chilies, minced

1 tablespoon ghee, melted

A pinch of salt and black pepper

1 teaspoon baking powder

2 eggs, whisked

½ cup chives, chopped

Directions:

In a bowl, mix the almond flour with the cream cheese, milk and the other Ingredients and whisk well.

Heat up the waffle iron, pour ¼ of the batter, cook for 6 minutes and transfer to a plate.

Repeat with the rest of the mix and Servings.

Nutrition: calories 273, fat 8, fiber 3.4, carbs 4.2, protein 8

Spicy curry chaffles

Preparation time: 10 minutes

Cooking time: 8 minutes

Servings: 4

Ingredients:

½ cup almond flour

½ cup coconut flour

1 tablespoon red curry paste

1 teaspoon hot paprika

1 red chili, minced

2 eggs, whisked

1 and ½ cups coconut milk

½ cup mozzarella, shredded

Directions:

In a bowl, mix the flour with the curry paste, eggs and the other Ingredients and whisk well.

Preheat the waffle iron, pour ¼ of the batter, cook for 8 minutes and transfer to a plate.

Repeat with the rest of the batter and Servings.

Nutrition: calories 263, fat 4.3, fiber 2.3, carbs 4, protein 8

Spicy salsa verde chaffles

Preparation time: 10 minutes

Cooking time: 8 minutes

Servings: 4

Ingredients:

1 cup coconut flour

1 cup coconut cream

2 tablespoons salsa verde

1 teaspoon cayenne pepper

¼ cup shallots, chopped

1/3 cup chives, chopped

½ cup mozzarella, shredded

2 eggs, whisked

A pinch of salt and black pepper

Directions:

In a bowl mix the flour with the cream, salsa verde and the other Ingredients and whisk well.

Heat up the waffle iron, pour ¼ of the batter and cook for 8 minutes.

Repeat with the rest of the salsa verde chaffle mix and Servings.

Nutrition: calories 263, fat 5.3, fiber 2.3, carbs 4, protein 4

Hot artichoke chaffles

Preparation time: 10 minutes

Cooking time: 10 minutes

Servings: 6

Ingredients:

1 cup coconut flour

1 cup cream cheese, soft

½ cup canned artichoke hearts, drained and chopped

2 red chilies, minced

1 teaspoon hot chili powder

1 teaspoon baking soda

2 eggs, whisked

½ cup coconut milk

2 zucchinis, grated

Directions:

In a bowl, mix the flour with the cheese, artichokes and the other Ingredients and whisk well.

Preheat the waffle iron, pour 1/6 of the batter, cook for 10 minutes and transfer to a plate.

Repeat with the rest of the chaffle batter and Servings them warm.

Nutrition: calories 282, fat 8.6, fiber 2.3, carbs 5, protein 8

Cake chaffle

Preparation time: 10 minutes

Cooking time: 8 minutes

Servings: 4

Ingredients: ¼ cup almond flour

2 eggs, whisked

2 tablespoons cream cheese, soft

2 tablespoons ghee, melted

½ teaspoon vanilla extract

½ teaspoon baking powder

2 tablespoons stevia ½ cup whipping cream

2 tablespoons swerve

½ teaspoon almond extract

Directions:

In a bowl, mix the flour with the eggs and the other Ingredients except the whipping cream, swerve and almond extract and whisk well.

Heat up the waffle iron, divide the batter into 4 parts, cook the chaffles one at the time and cool them down.

In a bowl, mix the remaining Ingredients and whisk well.

Layer the chaffles and the frosting mix and Servings the cake cold.

Nutrition: calories 140, fat 10.2, fiber 1, carbs 4.7, protein 4.7

Creamy vanilla cake chaffle

Preparation time: 10 minutes

Cooking time: 10 minutes

Servings: 2

Ingredients: 1 ounce cream cheese, soft

1 egg, whisked 2 tablespoons coconut flour

4 tablespoons heavy cream

2 teaspoons stevia

½ teaspoon vanilla extract

½ teaspoon cake batter extract

½ teaspoon baking soda

½ cup ghee, melted

½ cup swerve

Directions:

In a bowl, mix the cream cheese with the egg, 1 tablespoon heavy cream, flour, stevia, vanilla, cake batter extract and baking soda and whisk well. Heat up the waffle iron, pour half of the batter, cook for 10 minutes and transfer to a plate. Repeat with the rest of the batter and cool the chaffles down. In a bowl, mix the ghee with the remaining heavy cram and the other Ingredients and whisk.

Layer the chaffles and the frosting mix and Servings the cake.

Nutrition: calories 252, fat 9.3, fiber 2.3, carbs 12, protein 3.4

Coconut cake chaffle

Preparation time: 10 minutes

Cooking time: 10 minutes

Servings: 4

Ingredients:

3 tablespoons heavy cream

½ cup coconut cream

3 tablespoons cream cheese, soft

4 tablespoons coconut flour

1 tablespoon almond flour

4 eggs, whisked

1 teaspoon baking powder

2 tablespoons swerve

Directions:

In a bowl, mix the cream cheese with the flour and the other Ingredients except the coconut and heavy cream and whisk.

Heat up the waffle iron, pour ¼ of the batter, cook for 10 minutes and transfer to a plate.

Repeat with the rest of the batter and cool the chaffles down. In a bowl, mix the cream with the coconut cream and whisk.

Layer the chaffles and the coconut cream mix and Servings the cake cold.

Nutrition: calories 384, fat 32, fiber 3, carbs 23, protein 11

Lightning Source UK Ltd.
Milton Keynes UK
UKHW020641280621
386280UK00009B/512